FATIGUE: CAUSES, TREATMENT AND PREVENTION

Phylis A. Austin
Agatha M. Thrash, M.D.
Calvin L. Thrash, Jr, M.D.

Family Health Publications
8777 E. Musgrove Hwy.
Sunfield, MI. 48890

Table of Contents

FATIGUE

Everyone experiences fatigue at some time during his lifetime. Three out of four Americans complain of chronic fatigue according to a United States Public Health study. Fatigue is said to be the seventh most common complaint expressed in physician's offices in the United States. Today, fatigue cripples more people's lives than heart disease, arthritis, or bronchitis. It is the disease of our age. One would think that in this day of labor-saving devices fatigue would be rare, but in reality the opposite is true. Fatigue is more common today than it was 100 years ago when people worked much harder physically. Some early studies on fatigue have shown that it is far more common in individuals with a sedentary occupation than those who are physically active. Women complain of it more than men, probably because of less physical activity, improper dress, and poor nutrition. Fatigue is primarily a result of our lifestyles. An understanding of physiology and natural law will help many to conquer fatigue.

The causes of fatigue may be divided into two general classes: physiological and psychological. Psychological factors include boredom, stress, grief, anxiety, and depression. Physiological causes of fatigue are many. Table I shows some of the conditions known to cause or be associated with fatigue. We will focus on the most common of these.

Normal fatigue, which comes after a hard day of labor, is a blessing. It is our body's way of telling us it is time for rest. However, waking in the morning fatigued and hating the idea of facing the day is not the wish of anyone.

In this booklet we will consider some of the more common causes, prevention, and treatment of abnormal fatigue. If the control of fatigue leads us to a better lifestyle it will have been a blessing in disguise.

TABLE I: CAUSES OF FATIGUE

Alcoholism
Amyotrophic lateral sclerosis
Anemia
Arthritis
Asthma
Caffeinism
Chronic dehydration
Chronic obstructive
  pulmonary disease
Collagen-vascular disease
Congestive heart failure
Dementia
Diabetes mellitus
Drug use or abuse
Emphysema
Endocrine abnormalities
Environmental stress
Exercise, lack of
Fasting
Food allergy
Glomerulonephritis
Hepatitis
Hypertension
Hyperthyroidism
Hyperventilation
Hypoglycemia
Hypokalemia
Hypothyroidism
Inadequate rest
Infection
Infectious mononucleosis
Inflammatory bowel
  disease

Insomnia
Low cardiac output
Malignancy
Medications
Menorrhagia
Mitral valve
  dysfunction
Mononucleosis
Multiple sclerosis
Myasthenia gravis
Narcolepsy
Obesity
Parkinsonism
Peptic ulcer
Post-concussion
Pregnancy
Recent injury,
  illness, surgery
Rheumatic fever
Severe dietary
  restriction
Sickle cell
Sleep disturbance
Strep infections
Sydenham's chorea
Systemic lupus
Tension-fatigue syndrome
Tuberculosis
Undulant fever
Urinary tract infection
Ventilation, poor

ALLERGY AND FATIGUE

As early as 1873, Blackley wrote of allergy-induced fatigue. By 1930 Albert Rowe, M.D., enlarged on Blackley's observations and described patients suffering with weakness, lack of energy, sleepiness, irritability, fever, night sweats, chilling, depression, and body aches. That allergy and fatigue are associated is clearly pointed out by the term "allergic tension-fatigue syndrome." Symptoms are often vague and include muscle and bone pains, paleness, dark circles under the eyes, irritability and tension, headaches, stomachaches, and respiratory tract symptoms such as repeated "colds," asthma, or allergic rhinitis (hay fever), as well as fatigue. Bedwetting may be a problem and night sweats are sometimes observed.

Allergy-induced fatigue is typically present in the morning, despite a long night's sleep, or after an afternoon nap. Patients have difficulty awakening, or resist getting out of bed. The fatigue persists throughout the day, and may increase in the late afternoon and evening hours. Children suffering it may come in from play to lie down and rest, and may fall asleep in school despite adequate sleep the previous night. They may stop to rest if walking any distance; young children may wish to be carried. They may be very fidgety and restless. Ironically, these children may suffer from insomnia. Pale skin often persists, despite sun exposure. They may have puffiness about the face. Behavior may alternate between overactivity and lethargy. Activity and rest both seem to increase this type of fatigue. Laboratory studies for anemia may be negative, and the physician may be unable to find a physical cause for the child's symptoms. Even food allergy tests may be unrevealing. When the child is placed on a strict diet, free of the most common food allergens, symptoms may subside over a period of weeks.

Mental symptoms associated with the allergic tension-fatigue syndrome include irritability, mental confusion, obstinate behavior, temper tantrums, unhappiness, sluggish thinking, inability to concentrate, uncooperative, antisocial or rebellious behavior, emotional instability, unruliness, sullenness, nervousness and crying.

COMMON FOOD ALLERGENS
    Milk--Milk is the most common food allergen in the United States. Common sources of milk include whole, dried, skim, 2% milk, and buttermilk, custards, cheese, cream or creamed foods, yogurt, sherbet, iced milk, and ice cream. Traces of milk are found in butter, breads, and many commercially prepared foods. Examine all foods for milk products such as lactose, milk

solids, sodium caseinate, sodium lactate, milk fats and whey. Dr. Frederick Speer of the Speer Allergy Clinic says that all patients allergic to cow's milk are also allergic to goat's milk.

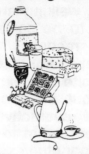

Kola--The kola nut family includes cola and chocolate. Both of these foods contain caffeine, as do coffee, tea, mate, cocoa and many soft drinks.

Corn--Corn syrup is used in the manufacture of nearly all chewing gum, candy, prepared meats (luncheon meats, sausages, wieners, bologna), many baked goods, canned fruits, and fruit juices, jams, jellies, sweetened syrups, pancake syrups, and ice cream. Hominy, grits, tortillas, Fritos®, burritos, tamales, and enchiladas contain corn. Cornstarch is often used as a thickener in soups and pies. Corn flour may be found in baked goods. Most American beer, bourbon, Canadian whiskey, and corn whiskey all contain corn. Corn oil should be avoided. Cornmeal is used in mush, scrapple, fish sticks, pancake, and waffle mixes.

Egg--Egg is capable of being such a potent allergen that even the odor of egg may produce symptoms. Many vaccines are egg-based. Baked goods, French toast, icings, meringue, candies, mayonnaise, salad dressings, meat

loaves, breaded foods, and noodles contain egg.
Legumes--Legumes (the pea family) include
peanut, soybean and licorice. Mature ("dry") peas
and beans are more likely to induce reactions
than are green or string beans, or green peas.
Many people sensitive to the legumes are also
allergic to honey, probably because in the United
States honey is gathered primarily from plants in
the legume family. Soybean concentrates are
common in baked goods, meats, and many
manufactured foods. Soybean oil is the most
commonly used oil in margarines, shortenings,
and salad oils. Peanuts are able to produce
severe reactions, including shock.

Citrus--Citrus fruits including oranges,
lemon, grapefruit, tangerine, and lime are
common allergens.

Apple--Apple is common in prepared foods.
Apple is found in apple vinegar, pickles, and
salad dressings.

Tomato--Tomato is found in meat loaf,
soups, stews, pizza, catsup, chili, salads, tomato
paste and juice, and many other prepared foods.
Potato, eggplant, tobacco, red and bell pepper,
cayenne, paprika, pimento and chili pepper are all
in the same family as tomato.

Grains--Wheat and small grains such as
rice, barley, oat, rye, millet, and wild rice may
induce allergic reactions. This group also
contains brown cane sugar, molasses, bamboo
shoots, and sorghum. Wheat is the most
allergenic; rye the least. Rye bread contains
more wheat flour than rye flour. Buckwheat is a
useful substitute for wheat.

Wheat is found in many dietary products,
including all baked goods, gravies, cream sauces,

macaroni, noodles, spaghetti, pie crusts, cereals, pretzels, chili, and breaded foods.

Food Additives and Spices--Spices and food additives often induce allergic reactions. Cinnamon is found in catsup, candies, chewing gums, cookies, cakes, chili, prepared meats, apple dishes, and pies. People who react to cinnamon usually react also to bay leaf. Pepper (black and white), cumin, basil, balm, horehound, marjoram, savory, rosemary, bergamot, coriander, sage, thyme, spearmint, peppermint and oregano often cause reactions.

Amaranth and tartrazine are possibly the artificial food colorings most likely to produce symptoms. They are common in carbonated beverages, breakfast drinks such as Tang® and Hi-C®, bubble gum, Popsicles®, Kool-Aid®, Jello®, and many medications.

Meats--Pork is the most common meat allergen, but oyster, clam, abalone, shrimp, crab, lobster, all true fish (such as tuna, salmon, catfish and perch), chicken, turkey, duck, goose, pheasant, quail, beef, veal, lamb, rabbit, squirrel, and venison may all induce symptoms.

Environmental Allergens

Individuals may be sensitive to environmental substances other than foods. Plants, molds, gases, animals and their hair, chemicals, drugs, cosmetics, synthetic fabrics, and a host of other factors may induce allergic reactions. Our energy supply is depleted with every reaction. A natural lifestyle, providing pure air, natural, additive-free foods, and a minimum of drug and chemical use may greatly reduce allergic reactions.

BLOOD SUGAR AND FATIGUE

High blood sugar levels (diabetes) or low blood sugar levels (hypoglycemia) may both lead to fatigue. In either case the body is unable to maintain proper blood sugar levels, which severely stresses the adrenal glands. The adrenal glands are basic to maintaining energy levels, and with the liver and pancreas, are responsible for producing hormones to keep the blood sugar level at the optimum level.

The two adrenal glands, one perched on top of each kidney, are endocrine glands. That

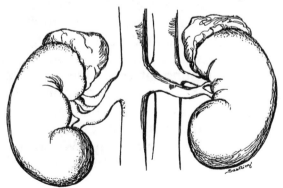

means that they produce and secrete hormones directly into the bloodstream. The hormones produced by the adrenals are essential to energy metabolism. The outer portion of the adrenals produce three different classes of hormones: glucocorticoids, mineralocorticoids, and sex hormones. Glucocorticoids are the hormones which function in the metabolism of carbohydrates, fats, and proteins, while mineralocorticoids regulate minerals, such as salt, potassium, and magnesium. Cortisol, one of the glucocorticoids, is essential to the liver in the regulation of blood sugar levels.

The inner portion of the adrenal gland produces catecholamines, adrenalin, and norepinephrine. These hormones function in the "fight or flight" response. A portion of the body's stress response includes raising the blood sugar to provide sufficient energy for the emergency. Any type of stress will induce production of these hormones; stress of prolonged duration will tax the adrenal glands. Overwork, overeating, high nutrient supplementation, lack of exercise, improper diet, and poor lifestyle habits tax the adrenal glands, decreasing their ability to function. People who use stimulants such as coffee, nicotine, or other chemical substances to push the adrenals to function above their normal level may cause adrenal exhaustion. Sugar, while not typically classified as a stimulant, has a temporarily stimulating effect. The pancreas is stimulated to secrete insulin in response to high blood sugar levels, and the insulin causes blood sugar to be absorbed into the cells, providing a sudden supply of fuel for energy. When the cells absorb all the sugar they can hold the additional sugar is placed in storage. Glycogen, the storage form of sugar, is deposited in the liver and muscles.

Such large amounts of insulin are produced in response to high blood sugar levels that sometimes the body overrreacts, and low blood sugar results. This leads to fatigue, which in turn, leads to a craving for more sugar to boost blood sugar levels. The cycle continues. The pancreas and liver become fatigued from attempting to control the blood sugar surges and dips.

The adrenals are responsible for mobilizing the energy-providing glycogen stored in the liver and muscles. Unfortunately, artificial stimulants may have already exhausted the adrenal glands and made them unable to function at their peak.

There is a natural stimulant for the adrenal glands--exercise!

Fatigue associated with low blood sugar is typically present on awakening in the morning, improves slightly after breakfast, and typically worsens in the midafternoon. Headache, weakness, sweating, dizziness, and fainting may be reported.

Fatigue present only in the morning may be due to poor bedroom ventilation, improper sleep, excessive stimulation of the senses--visual, sexual, or auditory-- or "cumulative fatigue" from long term stress or overwork.

Oral glucose tolerance tests are often not accurate in diagnosing hypoglycemic fatigue due to irregularities in glucose absorption. Some patients who suffer hypoglycemic fatigue demonstrate a flat curve on intravenous glucose tolerance testing. One study of a group of patients complaining of exhaustion and fatigue revealed that approximately one-third of them had decreased glucose tolerance.

HEALTH RECOVERY DIET

With proper diet and lifestyle the adrenals, pancreas, and liver may recover some of their ability to maintain blood sugar levels. The following program is suggested:

Avoid all refined sugars including white, brown, and raw sugar, fructose, honey, syrups, jams, jellies, preserves and Jello®. Pies, cakes, and sweetened desserts of any type should not be used. Make your own healthful desserts without sugar. A good vegetarian cookbook should have several recipes. Tests performed at the Brookhaven National Laboratory demonstrate that two to five percent more carbohydrate is converted to fat when persons are on a high sugar diet than when on a high unrefined carbohydrate diet.

Cheese, milk, and milk products are best eliminated. Milk contains leucine, which has been shown to induce hypoglycemic syndrome. Milk stimulates insulin secretion approximately five times greater than that expected from glucose.

Refined grains, including white breads, crackers, saltines, white macaroni, white rice, spaghetti, and other refined grain foods should be replaced with whole grain products.

Extremely sweet fruits such as raisins, dates, and figs are concentrated foods, and are best eliminated in severe cases for at least a year after beginning the diet. After a year small amounts may be introduced on a trial basis, and used if no symptoms develop. Bananas, watermelon, mangoes, and sweet potatoes are all in this category. Grapes and raisins may induce symptoms in some people.

Caffeine, nicotine, and alcohol are all harmful to the blood sugar regulating mechanisms of the body. Coffee, tea, cola drinks and chocolate all contain caffeine or caffeine-like substances. Many over-the-counter medications contain caffeine.

All soft drinks contain excessive amounts of sugar or sweeteners. This includes Kool-Aid®. Fruit juices are concentrated foods and should be used sparingly, if at all. It is much better to use the whole fruit.

Spices have an adverse effect on the nervous system and may aggravate symptoms. Vinegar and vinegar-containing foods may be prepared using lemon juice and salt in place of the vinegar.

PSYCHOLOGICAL CAUSES OF FATIGUE

The emotions may be the most powerful influences on the body. Fear, sorrow, guilt, and depression may as effectively depress body functions as a powerful drug. Anxiety, anger, resentment, bitterness, and frustration drain our energy. Sorrow and grief depress body functions, and sufferers often walk about with head hanging down and shoulders slumped. Their sorrow is like a heavy burden on their back. The slumped shoulders decrease lung expansion, while nature calls for a sigh to increase oxygen exchange in the lungs.

Joy induces dilation of the capillaries and arteries, increasing blood supply throughout the body. This change may stimulate activity such as "jumping for joy." The eyes become brighter, thinking becomes clearer, respirations deepened, heart beats become stronger, and digestion becomes more efficient. We now have some physiologic insight into the text "A merry heart doeth good like a medicine."

Fear may produce a loss of strength so severe as to cause paralysis. The individual may be unable to move, despite great danger. The blood vessels contract, causing the skin to become pale. The heart beats faster and with greater force. Goose pimples may rise, and the person may feel chilled. Eyes dilate and the person may lose bowel or bladder control as a result of action of the sympathetic nervous system.

Worry is a common source of fatigue, and is non-productive. Worry induces increased adrenalin secretion, which raises blood pressure. It has been shown to have pronounced effects on the thyroid, pancreas, and pituitary. The mental short-circuiting caused by worry drains energy which could be put to other more constructive purposes. Heavy intellectual work is less draining than negative emotions such as worry. The effects of worry are very similar to those of overwork. Worry increases the pulse rate, weakens muscle tone, induces lung congestion, causes paling of the skin, chills the extremities, and produces sleep disturbances. Exhaustion of the cranial nerves leads to pupil dilation. Blood pools in the internal organs because of the contraction of surface blood vessels. The worrier may break out in a cold sweat.

The person who worries constantly should learn to cast his cares on the Lord. Prayer may bring renewed physical, mental, and spiritual strength. Prayer brings divine strength in the form of courage and faith. Christ often spent the night in prayer without manifestations of fatigue.

Distraction is one of the best treatments for worry. When the attention is fully occupied with a wholesome subject, one cannot worry. Wood chopping, gardening, carpentry, and nature study are all excellent methods of mental diversion.

The worrier must also exercise his will in the cessation of worry. He must determine to turn his thoughts to other topics when he begins to worry. No one can eliminate worry as effectively as the worrier. An interest in the well-being of another individual or group of individuals is a worthwhile diversion.

Faith is the opposite of worry. The two cannot exist together. When tempted to worry, the Christian may turn to the Bible for comfort. Repeating and meditating on Bible texts will cast out worry. Here are a few suggestions:

"Be still and know that I am God." Ps 46:10

"Come unto me, all ye that labor, and are heavy laden and I will give you rest.

"Take my yoke upon you, and learn of me; for I am meek and lowly in heart: and ye shall find rest for your souls." Matt. 11:28-29.

"Wait on the Lord: be of good courage, and he shall strengthen thine heart." Ps 27:14

Boredom

Boredom in itself is an energy draining stress. Parents note that children who are too exhausted to do their household chores have an instant energy infusion when invited to go down to the corner lot for a softball game.

Lack of interest in the task at hand is fatiguing. We should cultivate the trait of being interested in whatever our duties may be. People who are uninterested in what they are doing are like a man trying to drive with his foot on the brake. Remember Solomon's advice: "Whatsoever

thy hand findeth to do, do it with all thy might."
Ecclesiastes 9:10.

Take up a new hobby, go to work a new
way, do something out of the ordinary to relieve
boredom. Half an hour of acute boredom can
use more nervous energy than you expend in a
whole day's work.

Compulsions

People who are compulsive often complain
of continuous fatigue. They feel that they cannot
relax until everything that needs to be done is
finished. They cannot stop until everything on
their list is complete, despite the fact that they
are weary.

Depression

Some eight million Americans are
depressed at any one time. Depression is often
expressed in the form of chronic fatigue which
may be overwhelming and make it difficult to
perform routine, simple tasks. Movement may be
slowed, and sleep disruptions are common.
There are two typical forms of sleep disturbance
in depression; the first is difficulty falling asleep,
the second, early awakening with inability to get
back to sleep.

Depression and fatigue are commonly seen
together. One writer estimates that 80% of all
patients seen in private medical practices show
signs of mild depression, with easy fatigability.
Some physicians who deal with these people
recognize a pattern that often characterizes them:
(1) Food sensitivities, (2) Inadequate water intake
and, (3) Inadequate exercise. The food allergies
cause dysfunction of the brain, made worse by

not having enough water to dilute the allergens which are kept in the body longer by impaired or slowed ciruclation due to little exercise.

Emotions

Negative emotions such as jealousy, resentment, anger, and hatred are all energy draining. Conversely, a sense of gratitude to the Lord for His constant blessings to us is a positive, energy-giving emotion.

Noise

Mental or physical stress drains the body's energy supply, leading to fatigue. Noise is often a source of stress. Television, radio, and high-fi's playing in the home may reduce one's ability to cope with the problems of daily life. Even the background noise in a city may be sufficient to induce fatigue. Country living may be helpful in eliminating this type of stress. Loud noises are fatiguing. A group of researchers at Bellevue Hospital in New York popped an inflated paper bag near the head of a group of patients. Brain pressure increased to four times normal whether the patient expected the noise or not. A second noise a few seconds later induced even greater increases in brain pressure. Noise may induce fatigue without the individual being aware of it. Both quality and quantity of work suffer under noisy conditions. A study at Colate University demonstrated that typists working in a noisy environment used 19% more energy than similar typists working in quiet circumstances.

Lack of Organization

Planning activities for the day enables one

to go from one task to another without the frustration of trying to decide what to do next.

Stress

Stress and fatigue have much in common and are often observed in the same individual. Exercise neutralizes stress. Dr. Hans Selye exposed ten unexercised rats to the stresses each of us are subjected to on a daily basis. Within a month every rat in the group was dead. A similar group of rats who were physically well-conditioned thrived despite being placed under the very same stresses. Activity, rather than inactivity, is recommended for individuals under stress.

Lack of balance in the lifestyle may be stressful. Using one part of the body to excess, as excessive mental work without balancing physical exercise, taxes the body. Hans Selye, whose name is synonymous with stress research, describes a general adaptation syndrome to stress. At first the body feels the stress, then reacts to it. If the stress is prolonged over a long period of time, the stress-reaction mechanisms become exhausted and unable to react any longer. Then the body's systems begin to break down one after the other--first an organ fails, then emotional or mental disorders follow. The process should be recognized early and correction instituted.

MISCELLANEOUS CAUSES OF FATIGUE

Anemia

Anemia is probably the physical condition most commonly associated with fatigue, but most fatigue is actually due to other causes. Some people have amazing energy and drive with very low hemoglobin levels. A slow drop in hemoglobin is less likely to produce symptoms of fatigue than a sudden drop, such as from a hemorrhage. Iron-deficiency anemia, particularly in menstruating women, may produce fatigue. The adult body holds roughly three to four grams of iron. The loss of a half teaspoon of blood causes about one milligram of iron to be lost. Persons who take aspirin may suffer anemia due to blood loss from the stomach. Women who suffer iron-deficiency anemia may benefit from iron supplements, but women who have only borderline anemia apparently do not. Two groups of mildly anemic women, treated with either placebo or iron therapy, demonstrated no significant differences in symptoms. Women who constantly diet in an attempt to have a slim figure so cherished in today's society are particularly prone to inadequate nutrition, which in turn, leads to fatigue. Hemoglobin carries oxygen to all parts of the body. When levels are low the body is not so well supplied with oxygen. Very high hemoglobin levels may also produce fatigue. For persons with high hemoglobin, donating blood may increase energy levels.

Blood Pressure
Low or high blood pressure may contribute to fatigue. Outdoor exercise is the best treatment for low blood pressure.

Constipation
Constipation produces a feeling of fatigue in some people. Lack of adequate fluid intake, insufficient exercise, improper diet, drug use, poor posture, and mental factors may contribute to constipation. Putrefaction, which produces fatigue-inducing toxins, is more pronounced in individuals who use large amounts of eggs and meat. Putrefactive bacteria thrive on animal protein.

Dehydration
Dehydration is often a cause of fatigue. A lack of water reduces work performance more rapidly than a lack of food. A study reported in the *American Journal of Physiology* demonstrated a very real relationship between water intake and energy. A group of athletes were exercised on a treadmill for as long as possible without taking any water. They were able to continue walking

for about 3 1/2 hours. After a few days of recovery time, the same men were again placed on the treadmill, but were given as much water to drink as they wanted. They were able to walk about six hours on this day.

HYDRATION AND EXERCISE TOLERANCE

▨▨▨▨
No water

▨▨▨▨▨▨
Water as desired

▨▨▨▨▨▨▨▨ +
Replacement of lost water

On the third trial the men were required to drink enough water to replace what they were losing in perspiration. They were still walking, and felt they could go on indefinitely, at seven hours when the test was concluded. The study suggests that thirst is not an adequate guide to water requirements. These men were losing one-third more water than they were taking in when they drank as much as they wished. Fatigue may be due to the inability of the body to maintain adequate blood pressure in the absence of sufficient fluid. Simply refilling the blood vessels may be adequate to relieve this fatigue. Even the physical fitness of highly trained athletes will not overcome the fatigue of dehydration in sporting events. High humidity and high temperatures increase fluid loss, inducing quicker fatigue if adequate water is not taken. Water is the best substance to replace body fluids. Drinks commonly used by athletes are not so quickly absorbed by the body, and may induce electrolyte imbalance if used in excess. In some cases they actually worsen the tissue level dehydration.

Some people cannot tell the body's call for water from a call for food, and so they eat instead of drink. This increases the total caloric intake which leads to obesity. When you think you are hungry, taking a large glass of water may be sufficient to control the desire for food. If food is taken, even more water is actually required to dissolve the nutrients and transport them in the blood. Most people are chronically far behind in their water drinking because of the use of too much food.

Improper Dress

Tight shoes, collars, and corsets and girdles which constrict body organs and hinder proper breathing may contribute to fatigue. Clothing should allow for full and easy respiration and movement. The constant irritation of overly tight clothing can send up a barrage of sensory impulses that weary the poor brain.

Drug Use

Many drugs, alcohol, and other stimulants may cause malaise and tiredness. Tobacco is a common cause of fatigue. Dr. Harry Segal, of the University of Rochester School of Medicine and Dentistry, reported the cure of fatigue in several patients by simply persuading them to stop smoking. A number of studies demonstrate that non-smokers perform better than smokers on physical fitness studies.

A study from Switzerland reveals that smoking causes a loss of energy. Young adults who usually smoked 24 cigarettes a day had 10 percent more energy available for profitable activities on a day they did not smoke. Smoking induced a 20 percent increase in the heart rate and a 45 percent increase in production of the stress hormone, norepinephrine. Nicotine causes constriction of peripheral blood vessels, hindering blood flow. Lung capacity is reduced, decreasing blood oxygenation and an increased pulse rate forces the heart to work harder. Tobacco smoke contains about 4 percent carbon monoxide, a substance which hinders oxygen transport. Nicotine increases cerebral arousal and the pulse rate. A comparison of the sleep of smokers and non-smokers demonstrated that smokers took longer to get to sleep initially, and woke more frequently during the night. When the smokers stopped smoking, they fell asleep more quickly and slept more during the night.

Many drugs, including amphetamines, hypnotics, sedatives, sleeping pills, antihistamines, anticonvulsants, salicylates, analgesics, tetracyclines, birth control pills, adrenocorticosteroids, insulin, digitalis, some vitamin supplements, antidepressants, diuretics, and some blood pressure medications, are known to induce fatigue. Codeine-containing cough medications may induce fatigue as effectively as they control coughs. Many other drugs probably have similar effects.

Thousands of Americans walk about in

drug-induced stupors. They do not consider the fact that a drug with the power to control one symptom has the ability to change other metabolic activities. A study carried out in South Wales revealed that drug-induced fatigue was the third most common type of fatigue, more common than fatigue due to anemia, cancer, diabetes, or thyroid abnormalities.

Coffee, vitamin supplements, alcohol and sleeping pills are at best only a temporary solution to fatigue, and at worst are counter-productive. Habitual alcohol users often begin the day tired, perhaps due to malnutrition. Alcohol-induced liver damage hinders the proper handling of toxins and interferes with blood sugar control. Alcohol use interferes with the important REM (rapid-eye movement) sleep phases, and produces chronic sleep disturbances.

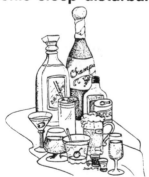

Environment

The physical environment may contribute to fatigue. Cluttered and messy working quarters and lack of elbow room may be more tiring than overwork. White colors are fatiguing, as are purple, brown, orange, and even some shades of blue. Medium green and yellow are restful colors. Glare off glass and metal tables may induce fatigue.

Stuffy, overheated rooms are tiring to both mind and body. The body reduces internal heat generation in response to external temperatures and becomes less active. Blood is pulled into the skin, depriving the internal organs of the blood which carries life-giving oxygen. A daily cold shower stimulates circulation and respiration and may increase metabolism 80 percent. Furthermore, a cold shower tones up the blood vessel muscles. With a high environmental temperature the blood vessels become weak and sluggish, but cold exposure causes them to contract to reduce the cooling of the blood. These "artery exercises" assist the blood vessels to maintain a healthy tone. Finish off your daily cold shower with a brisk towel rubdown.

Lack of Exercise

Lack of exercise, along with its almost invariable companion, inadequate water intake, is probably the most common cause of fatigue in the United States. We are a sedentary society. People are tired after a long day behind a desk and neglect to exercise, but if they would exercise, they would be amazed at how refreshed they feel afterwards. The exercise of mind and body must be properly balanced. Fatigue is largely a disease of those who work mainly with their minds. Those who use their muscles in their work do not tire as easily as those whose work is chiefly mental. Muscles have a greater capacity for work without fatigue than does the mind.

People whose work is primarily mental often become more fatigued than those with work of a physical nature. Only four hours' sleep is required to restore physical energy, but it may require twice that long to restore mental energy. To do mental work with a minimum of fatigue, be certain that there is an adequate supply of fresh air to ensure that the brain receives sufficient oxygen. A brisk walk may increase blood circulation to the brain 20 percent, resulting in clearer, more creative thinking. Without an active, healthy body, one cannot have a healthy mind.

Many think of jogging when they think of exercise and hesitate to begin an exercise program because they feel they can't jog. Dr. George Sheehan, a cardiologist and author of a book on running, states that in his opinion jogging is not necessary to a fitness program and that a brisk walk is as effective as jogging. Jogging does carry with it significant risk of injury according to a Centers for Disease Control study, which reports that in a 12-month period one-third of runners who jog six or more miles on a weekly basis will suffer an injury severe enough to force modification of their running program.

Physical activity is a very effective treatment for fatigue. Rest is not the solution for the fatigue resulting from poor physical conditioning. Slow circulation decreases the ability of the body to eliminate the toxic waste products of metabolism. Inactivity is often the real basis of fatigue--think how tired you are on Monday morning after a weekend of "rest." People who exercise regularly need less oxygen to perform the same amount of work as a man who spends his life in inactivity.

A group of 30 children seen at an Air Force hospital with complaints of fatigue were given a most unusual prescription. The doctors ordered that the children not watch any television at all. The symptoms vanished within two to three weeks in every child who was kept strictly on the program. Those who continued to watch television but on a more limited basis, had a reduction in symptoms, but not a complete remission.

Standing can be fatiguing, as lymph fluids and blood tend to accumulate in the legs. Walking causes contraction of the leg muscles which forces these fluids back up into the circulatory system.

Some feel that aging is more the result of inactivity than of passing years. We tend to reduce our activities as we age, which in turn causes us to become less fit.

The world champion weightlifter has no more muscles than an infant--his are just more developed. Studies show that a muscle contracted to two-thirds of its maximum ability and held in the contracted position for only six seconds once a day will acquire its maximum potential strength.

Physical fitness improves aerobic power and heat regulation, increases glycogen stores, and improves strength and posture, all of which decrease fatigue. Hans Selye, in his book, *The Stress of Life,* recommends short periods of physical activity which lead to acute fatigue as a treatment for chronic fatigue. Rest will relieve the acute fatigue and chronic fatigue will be lessened. Stress-induced fatigue is greatly helped by physical exercise, as is the depression often associated with fatigue.

Infections

Low-grade infections may produce chronic fatigue. They may persist for weeks after an episode of flu or other viral infection. The reasons for such occurrences are not yet understood, but they may be due to a change in the way muscles obtain their energy supply. Low grade infection of the urinary tract, prostate, sinuses, gums, throat, or skin may be present without the victim being aware of them. Keeping the body's immune system at its peak level by the use of a low sugar, low fat, vegetarian diet, exercise, and rest will assist the body in fighting off these infections.

Lead

"Get the lead out," is a common expression thrown at lazy or slowly moving individuals. Fatigue is an early manifestation of lead poisoning. Even low body lead levels may lead to fatigue. Common sources of lead exposure include leaded gasoline exhaust fumes, food, water, and air. Lead may be found in powdered bonemeal taken as a calcium supplement. When lead is consumed by animals, it is stored in the bones. Calcium supplements made from these bones may contain toxic levels of lead. Lead-containing food vessels, lead pottery glazes, and pesticides may yield toxic levels, and shellfish in contaminated waters may concentrate lead. Cow's milk and muscle meat may be lead sources, as may contaminated drinking water, cigarette smoke, and polluted air.

Overstimulation

From the time we open our eyes in the morning until we are asleep that night, we are bombarded by sensory stimulation--noise, lights, crowds, and vibrations. These are all energy-draining. At the end of the day we may be tired from over-stimulation rather than overwork. We come home exhausted, prop our feet up, and turn on the television for still more sensory stimulation.

Overarousal and overstimulation are energy costly. In our society we are constantly bombarded with sexually arousing movies, television programs, magazines, books, and billboards. Some types of entertainment enjoyed by teenagers are overstimulating and energy draining.

Excessively spicy foods stimulate the taste buds to excess. This overstimulation robs us of the ability to enjoy the simple things of life. Excessive stimulation of the emotions needs to be constantly and carefully guarded against. Excessive marital relations, eating too much, and any normal and necessary sensory stimulation which proceeds to the point of being excessive can cause tiredness.

Overweight

Being overweight puts an extra load on the circulatory and muscular systems of the body, hastening fatigue. The letters f-a-t are the first three letters in the word "fatigue." Isaac Stern observes that fat people are usually tired people. Carrying around a lot of extra weight is certain to make one tired.

People who are overweight are required to

carry a heavy load with them everywhere they go. The typical American male who is 20 pounds overweight uses about 14 percent more energy to move about than does a man of normal weight. The heart must pump blood to supply oxygen to the additional tissue, and exercise is typically avoided by the overweight person. A study by Dr. Jean Mayer, a Harvard University nutritionist, revealed that overweight teenagers often ate less than slimmer peers, but were less physically active. They spent about four times as much time in sedentary activities (reading and watching television) as did the slimmer comparison group, and exercised only about one-third as much. Further, when they did exercise, they did it with less vigor and energy than their slimmer peers.

Resolve to lose excess pounds and use the energy for more profitable activities. Obesity is more often caused by lack of activity than by overeating. Reducing caloric intake produces a slowing of the metabolic rate, hindering weight loss. Furthermore, muscle tissue is lost along with fat. Exercise increases the metabolic rate, resulting in more effective burning of calories, while it builds up muscles and aids in appetite control.

Overweight persons are often hindered in their breathing because of fat collected around the abdomen. This fat hinders movement of the diaphragm, decreasing the amount of air which can be pulled into the lungs.

Poor Posture

Poor posture leads to fatigue in several ways. The first is that slouching reduces the ability of the lungs to exchange air. Oxygen is not carried to the cells of the body so efficiently; waste products are not eliminated so readily. Waste products are toxins which produce fatigue. The heart must work harder to pump blood through the cramped lungs. At rest about half of our total blood supply is in our abdominal organs. Blood flow may be increased about one-third with proper posture. With poor posture the abdominal organs are displaced and pushed into abnormal position, hindering their circulation and function. Blood vessels are displaced, slowing blood flow.

Poor posture places a tax on the muscles, tendons, ligaments, and bones of the body by forcing them to hold the body in an unnatural position. When the head, which weighs about 10 pounds, is balanced over the shoulders, the muscles have to work very little to maintain head position, but when the head is bent forward the muscles must contract to prevent the head from falling down on the chest. A constant poor posture produces permanent strain on muscles and ligaments, resulting in a significant energy expenditure. Remember at all times to maintain good posture, whether standing, sitting, or lying.

Pregnancy
Fatigue is a common symptom of pregnancy. Although this fatigue cannot be prevented it may be minimized by regular out-of-doors exercise. Do not overdo exercise, but exercises such as brisk walking are helpful. Even rocking in a rocking chair will improve circulation.

Coffee, tea, soft drinks, and other stimulants should be avoided as they may be harmful to your infant. Sweets may give a temporary lift, but provide empty calories which will take the place of nutritious foods.

Accept the fact that your first responsibility is to your unborn child. Set aside social obligations to assure adequate rest. Bedtime should be regular seven days a week. Even if you have difficulty sleeping, quiet rest is helpful. Frequent 10 minute rest breaks may help you get through the day. Do not lie for long periods on the back as the heavy uterus will fall against the large blood vessels behind it, and impede circulation. The ideal sleep position is on the side.

Premenstrual Syndrome (PMS)

Premenstrual syndrome may produce fatigue. Much of this fatigue can be eliminated by proper exercise, diet, and rest.

Lack of Rest

Sleep deficiency is a frequent cause of the fatigue prevalent in today's society. Anyone who burns the candle at both ends is going to suffer fatigue. Regular, restful sleep is essential to an abundant energy supply. The duties of the day should not take up the sleeping hours. Poorly rested individuals expend three times more energy accomplishing a task than do well-rested persons.

Insomnia often leads to fatigue, but some simple steps may go far in preventing sleep loss. Sleeping pills should be avoided, as their effect may make a person lethargic for 18-24 hours.

Caffeine-containing beverages are known to disrupt sleep and should be eliminated. It is not entirely the caffeine, as decaffeinated drinks disrupt sleep and contain naturally-occurring chemicals that injure the nervous system.

Outdoor exercise is productive of good sleep. Timing of the exercise, however, influences sleep. A study at Boston's Downstate Medical Center demonstrated that sleep is lighter on nights when no exercise is taken, and heaviest when exercise was performed in the afternoon. Evening exercise induced less sound sleep, probably acting as a stimulant.

An established bedtime routine, followed faithfully, is often helpful in getting to sleep. It may involve bathing, reading, Bible study and prayer, or other activities, but should be performed in the same manner every evening. The body becomes trained to go to sleep after the routine.

Some people report that a very effective treatment for insomnia is to try to stay awake. German physicians advise their insomnia patients to lie in bed and try to keep their eyes open as long as possible. The eyes become tired, and the lid-closing reflex leads to sleep. Warming the eyes with a wool scarf laid gently over the eyes may induce sleep.

Henry Ford, Sr., states that a day of rest is essential. "We would have had our Model A car in production six months sooner, if I had forbidden my engineers to work on Sunday," Ford said. "It took us all week to straighten out the mistakes they made on the day when they should have rested."

On the other hand, excessive sleep may be fatiguing. The typical adult probably needs seven to eight hours of sleep nightly, but individual needs vary and even one person may have different needs at different times. A syndrome of unclear thinking, difficulty getting started, and feelings of fatigue and lethargy has been associated with sleeping late, particularly if the individual has slept ten or more hours. The syndrome may persist for four to five hours, preventing the accomplishment of much during the day. The person who sleeps in on the weekend to catch up may be more tired than when he went to bed on Friday night. This points up the importance of regular bed and rising times every day of the week.

People who suffer sleep apnea (cessation of breathing) often complain of daytime fatigue. Overweight people who suffer sleep apnea are often benefited by weight loss.

Irregular Schedule

The body operates most efficiently on a regular schedule. It learns to produce various hormones at specific times in the 24 hour cycle in response to the body's needs at that time. Digestive fluids are produced when a meal is expected; to force the body to produce these substances on an irregular schedule taxes the body. Irregularity in meals also produces irregular blood sugar levels. Regular bed and rising times train the body to sleep and awaken at specific times. Both body and mind operate best on a regular schedule. Deviation from this schedule may be a fatigue-induced stress.

Lack of Sunlight

Sunlight exposure is essential to maximum energy levels. London zoo officials observed that some animals deprived of ultraviolet rays became sluggish and inactive. When provision was made for a more natural type of light, the animals perked up and became more active. Children grow faster during months with maximum hours of sunshine.

Thyroid

Individuals whose thyroids are under- or over-active may suffer chronic fatigue. An overactive thyroid may increase the metabolism, which burns energy supplies, and induces fatigue. Fatigue associated with an overactive thyroid generally comes on a few hours after getting up in the morning and is sometimes associated with muscle weakness. Metabolism is slowed with insufficient thyroid hormone, which produces fatigue. Thyroid testing is easy and accurate, involving blood tests available through a physician.

Toxins

Vinegar, pepper, mustard, and other condiments have a toxic effect on the body, forcing the body to expend energy to clear them from the tissues. Some of them have been shown to have an influence on metabolism. Indole and skatole, (products of putrefaction) found in cheese, are also toxins, and are known to be potent fatigue producers.

Car exhaust fumes are a source of carbon monoxide, which when inhaled decreases the body's ability to transport oxygen.

Insecticides and radioactivity are both reported to cause fatigue. Fluorides, mercury, cadmium and copper may cause fatigue.

Inadequate Ventilation

Breathing poor air decreases energy performance. A study of men lifting dumbbells demonstrated better performance in fresh air than in stagnant air. Fresh air in the bedroom is particularly important. A good supply of oxygen in the lungs and blood cells is essential to high energy levels.

People who spend hours slumped over their work tend to breathe shallowly, with resulting poor oxygen exchange which leads to fatigue. Deep breathing is essential for mental workers--studies suggest that memory may be improved up to seven percent by deep breathing.

Humans can go for weeks without food, days without water, but only minutes without oxygen. Every cell of the body requires oxygen, which it obtains from the approximately 35 pounds of air we inhale each day.

Exercise is the best available respiratory stimulant. Even people who suffer from lung disease benefit by an exercise program. Increasing oxygen uptake increases energy levels.

Free respiration is hindered by obesity. Over half of our lung expansion is produced by the action of the diaphragm, a muscle which divides the chest from the abdomen. The diaphragm pushes the stomach and intestines down to allow lung expansion. Fat hinders this action.

Much of the fatigue common today is due to "lazy lung syndrome." Our lungs are not forced to work to capacity because of our sedentary lifestyle, and lose their ability to function to their potential.

Emotions play a significant role in our breathing. Our demonstrations of emotion-- laughter, gasps, crying, yelling--are all modified forms of breathing. We often attempt to control our breathing in an attempt to hide our emotions.

Sedentary workers should give attention to their breathing patterns, attempting to breathe deeper and more slowly. The base and apex of the lungs are brought into activity with deep respirations.

The brain uses almost one-fourth of our total oxygen uptake and cannot function effectively without an adequate supply of air.

FATIGUE IN CHILDREN

An epidemic of fatigue seems to have overcome American children. Parents can do much to eliminate the causes of this problem and help their children obtain the best possible start in life.

The typical child suffering from fatigue eats little or no breakfast. If he does eat breakfast the foods are sugar-laden, rather than whole grains. If he becomes hungry by midmorning, he is given a snack which is usually something sweet. The midday meal is not eaten well because the midmorning snack has destroyed the appetite, but an afternoon snack is demanded.

Parents should expect a child to eat a generous breakfast of fruit and whole grains. No refined sugar should be given to the child, particularly a child with a poor appetite. If he refuses to eat breakfast he should not be force-fed, but should be told that he will have to wait until time for the midday meal. At that meal he should be given vegetables and whole grains, without any sugar. Again, if the meal is not eaten he should be instructed that he must wait until the next meal. Absolutely nothing but pure, fresh water should be allowed between meals for a child over age three. The digestive organs need time to rest, and eating between meals keeps them constantly laboring, which often uses up more energy than it provides.

The use of milk should be studied. Many children are allergic to milk, and milk often destroys the appetite for fruits and vegetables which do not cause a problem.

After the age of two or three years most children do best on a two meal a day program, eliminating supper. It is known that heavy suppers interfere with restful, refreshing sleep, an essential factor in fighting fatigue.

Television and sedentary activities should be limited. Many children are tired from the lack of physical exercise and the mental stimulation that comes from hours of television watching. Out-of-doors exercise, particularly working with their parents in useful labor such as lawn care, gardening, and similar activities, is far more beneficial than television. The child's social activities should be carefully supervised. Competition in games should be avoided; activities should be planned which teach cooperation rather than competition. Contests are stressful.

Bedtime and rising time should be the same 365 days a year. Holidays, vacations, and weekends are not reason for deviation. The child who knows that he must go to bed at a certain time puts up less fuss than the child who knows that when he fusses he will be allowed to stay up later. Fresh air should be abundant in the bedroom, and as much time as possible spent out-of-doors during the day. The child should not be permitted to waste the early morning hours in bed. After adequate sleep he should be expected to be up and about the activities of the day.

Food allergies are a common cause of fatigue in children. See the chapter on food allergies and fatigue in the book, *Food Allergies Made Simple,* for further information on this topic.

THE ANTI-FATIGUE DIET

The Stress and Hypertension Clinics at the United States Naval Weapons Plant developed what they call an "anti-stress diet." Irritants (tobacco, spices), stimulants (tea, coffee), and depressants (alcohol, drugs) were prohibited. The free use of whole-grain foods, fruits and vegetables was encouraged. They report that the results were "most gratifying," with an improvement in the general health of the people on the diet.

Overeating, eating between meals, and eating heavy suppers may all lead to fatigue. Heavy suppers have been shown to interfere with refreshing sleep. A good breakfast is essential to high energy levels during the day. Dr. Samuel Arnold of Morristown, New Jersey, observed that 88 percent of women who complained of fatigue ate a poor breakfast; and, when instructed in a proper diet, reported increased energy levels.

The two-meal-a-day plan is a great energy conserver. The body expends vast amounts of energy producing the enzymes necessary for food digestion. Since it requires four to five hours to digest a meal, the three-meal-a-day plan keeps the body expending digestive energy most of the working day. The two-meal plan allows the stomach rest periods during the day. While the rest may not seem significant when considered on the basis of one day, it becomes significant when considered over a period of weeks, months, or years. The early Greeks and Romans, both renowned as athletes, ate only two meals a day. Today, the long-lived Hunzas eat only one or two meals a day, and often fast. Some observers point out that the three-meal-a-day plan prevails in countries that use a lot of refined foods.

One simple principle is basic to the anti-fatigue diet: eat a wide variety of healthful foods in their natural, unrefined states. Individual meals should be composed of three or four foods; the next meal should be composed of different foods to obtain variety. A great variety at one meal is neither necessary nor beneficial.

Foods high in sugar and fat are stressors to the body, requiring it to expend energy to handle them. Concentrated foods, including vitamin and mineral supplements, may induce fatigue by taxing the gastrointestinal system. A study reported in 1942 revealed that men on a high fat diet fatigued quicker and were less efficient.

Overeating is a tax upon the body and may induce fatigue. Eat enough to satisfy hunger, but not necessarily appetite. The act of metabolizing excess food is an unnecessary tax upon the body energies. Stomach stretching caused by over-eating may interfere with the function of the diaphragm, making breathing more difficult, and diminishing the supply of oxygen available to the body.

Rich foods are a similar burden. Many people hate Mondays because of overly rich, stimulating food eaten over the weekend, and a reduction in their normal levels of physical activity. A heavy noon meal leads to afternoon fatigue, as blood is drawn into the gastrointestinal tract to deal with the food.

A vegetarian diet is known to produce greater physical stamina. When one gives up meat he may suffer a temporary loss of energy because of the stimulatory effect of the meat, but he will soon recover and will be amazed at the increase in stamina if he also adopts a good lifestyle. A person who is considering adopting a vegetarian diet often becomes concerned that he will lose strength when he stops eating meat. Elephants and horses are vegetarians, but are well-known for their strength.

Waste products, such as lactic acid, produced by body activity, produce fatigue. The blood must be alkaline in order to neutralize this acid and prevent fatigue. Alkaline foods, mainly fruits and vegetables, keep the blood alkaline. Even after fatigue, the vegetarian recovers five times faster than the meat eater. Too much protein, especially protein of animal origin, may make a person tired. Meat contains urinary or fatigue wastes. These waste products are not found in proteins of vegetable origin.

Iron-deficiency anemia is a frequent cause of fatigue. Raisins, whole grains, prunes, and green leafy vegetables are good sources of iron. Cast-iron cookware imparts iron to the food cooked in it, particularly if the food is high in acid, such as tomatoes. A tablespoon of blackstrap molasses contains 3.2 milligrams of iron. Iron absorption may be decreased if tea or coffee is taken with the meal. The heavy use of alcohol hinders red blood cell formation. Iron is best absorbed in an acid environment, so antacids decrease iron absorption by neutralizing the normally acid stomach.

Table II shows the iron value of some common foods.

Vitamin Supplements

Some have advocated the use of vitamin supplements in the treatment of fatigue, but the treatment is controversial. At least one report in the medical literature has suggested that vitamin E induces fatigue. About a week after beginning the intake of 800 I.U. of vitamin E daily, a California physician suffered fatigue, weakness, and flu-like symptoms. He stopped the vitamin, and symptoms subsided. Thinking he had had the flu, he resumed the vitamin intake and symptoms reappeared. He had been advising many of his patients to take vitamin E, and many of them reported similar experiences and had to cease the supplement use.

Studies showing benefit from vitamin supplements were probably done with patients who had acute vitamin deficiencies. Doctors Ancel Keys and Austin Henschel studied the possibility of "vitamin supercharging" in the prevention of fatigue. Their studies showed that healthy, normal men do not benefit from vitamin supplements.

A similar study evaluated the B vitamins in

TABLE II: IRON CONTENT OF FOODS

FOOD	IRON MG
Almonds, 3 1/2 oz.	4.7
Apricots, raw 3 1/2 oz.	.5
Avocado, Calif. 3 1/2 oz.	.6
Beet greens, cooked 1/2 cup	1.90
Black-eyed peas, cooked 3 1/2 oz.	2.1
Broccoli, raw, 1 stalk	1.10
Brussels sprouts, 6-8 med, cooked	1.10
Cashews, 3 1/2 oz.	3.8
Cauliflower, 1 cup, raw	1.10
Chard, cooked, 3/5 cup	1.80
Corn meal, 1 cup	2.92
Cowpeas, mature, cooked 3 1/2 oz.	1.30
Currants, raw, 3 1/2 oz.	1.1
Dandelion greens, cooked, 3 1/2 oz.	1.80
Elderberries, raw, 3 1/2 oz.	1.6
Endive, raw, 20 leaves	1.70
Figs, dried, 3 1/2 oz.	3.0
Garbanzo beans, dry, 3 1/2 oz.	6.9
Green beans, cooked, 3 1/2 oz.	.6
Jerusalem artichoke, raw, 4 small	3.40
Kale, cooked, 3 1/2 oz.	1.60
Kidney beans, red, cooked, 1/2 c.	3.33
Lentils, cooked, 3 1/2 oz.	2.1
Lima beans, green, cooked, 5/8 c.	2.50
Lima beans, mature, boiled 3 1/2 oz	3.1
Mustard greens, cooked, 1/2 c.	1.80
Parlsey, raw, 3 1/2 oz.	6.20
Peach, raw, 3 1/2 oz.	.5
Peanuts, raw	2.1
Peas, raw, 3 1/2 oz.	.3
Pecans, 3 1/2 oz.	2.4
Pistachio, 3 1/2 oz.	7.3
Potato, white, baked, 3 1/2 oz.	.7
Prunes, dried, 3 1/2 oz.	3.9
Pumpkin seeds, 3 1/2 oz.	11.2
Raisins, 3 1/2 oz.	3.5
Rice bran, 100 grams	16.1
Romaine lettuce, raw, 3 1/2 oz.	1.40
Rye, 3 1/2 oz.	3.7
Sesame seeds, whole, 3 1/2 oz.	10.5
Soybean flour, defatted, 3 1/2 oz.	11.1
Soybeans, immature, cooked, 2/3 c.	2.50
Soybeans, mature, cooked, 1/2 c.	2.70
Spinach, raw, 3 1/2 oz.	3.1
Strawberries, raw, 3 1/2 oz.	1.0
Squash, acorn, 3 1/2 oz.	1.0
Squash, butternut, baked, 1/2 cup	1.60
Squash, hubbard, baked, 1 cup	1.60
Sweet potato, 1 large, baked	1.60
Turnip greens, cooked, 2/3 cup	1.10
Walnuts, 3 1/2 oz.	6.0
Wheat, 3 1/2 oz.	3.5

the prevention of fatigue. This study also revealed that individuals who have adequate nutrition do not benefit from supplements of vitamin B complex. Even slight deviations from a wholesome diet, if continued over prolonged periods of time, takes its toll on energy levels.

Refined foods do not contain many of the nutrients essential for abundant energy. Deficiencies of magnesium, calcium, iron, potassium and iodine are all associated with fatigue, and these substances are often not present in refined foods.

Calcium deficiency may produce fatigue far greater than one would expect in proportion to the amount of activity performed. Further, it may induce insomnia, which increases fatigue. Whole grain bread is a good source of calcium. Enriched white bread contains less calcium than whole grains. Green vegetables are another good source of calcium.

Low magnesium levels are known to contribute to fatigue. Taking antacids containing aluminum reduces available magnesium. Refining foods removes much of this energy-producing mineral. Foods high in magnesium include whole grains, green vegetables, and nuts. A diet high in sugar induces magnesium deficiency. Magnesium is a part of chlorophyll, the green coloring matter found in plants.

Women who take calcium supplements may create an imbalance in their calcium-magnesium ratio, leading to poor absorption of magnesium.

Potassium is essential for proper muscle function, and without adequate supplies we suffer decreased muscle strength and tone. Many fruits and vegetables, including celery, bananas, oranges, parsley, carrots, potatoes, and tomatoes, are excellent sources of potassium. Refined carbohydrates such as sugar, tend to cause potassium loss, as does the use of diuretics, soft drinks, coffee and tea. Salt interferes with the sodium-potassium balance of the body, producing energy-draining fluid retention. Use salt sparingly and avoid highly salted foods such as pickles and potato chips.

Large amounts of sugar may cause a reduction of the potassium in the blood, which leads to weakness or even paralysis.

Laxatives such as Epsom salts and other magnesium salts cause both water and potassium loss, which may induce weakness and fatigue.

Low levels of vitamin C may be associated with fatigue. Fresh, raw fruits and vegetables supply vitamin C. Broccoli, kale, and parsley contain twice as much vitamin C as oranges. To preserve vitamin C during preparation, foods should be lightly cooked in a small amount of water, with the minimum possible preparation. Cooking, dicing, and shredding all destroy vitamin C. Foods kept warm for prolonged periods lose much vitamin C. Fatigue is a symptom of scurvy, a vitamin C deficiency, and may be present six to eight weeks before clinical signs of scurvy appear.

High vitamin C levels increase the amount of glycogen (the energy-storage substance) in the liver, and muscles, thus delaying fatigue.

Natural Treatments for Fatigue

Some safe, effective treatments may be helpful until you can locate and eliminate the cause of your fatigue.

Set side a regular time each day for prayer, Bible study, and communion with the Creator. This will be a potent stress reliever.

Deep breathing exercises improve the oxygen supply to the brain, and in turn, to the entire body. Standing upright, hands on the hips, in a well-ventilated room, or out-of-doors, take deep, slow breaths, as if to fill the lungs from the bottom up. Take as complete a breath as possible, hold for the count of 20, exhale completely and hold for a count of ten. This may be repeated 20-40 times, three times a day.

Ice-cold foot baths are stimulating. Sit on the edge of the tub and run cold water over your feet and ankles. As your tolerance for cold increases, add ice cubes to a tub of water two to four inches deep and place your feet in the ice water for 30 seconds to three minutes. Dry the feet well after removing them from the water. The feet should be warm before the foot bath is begun. Rubbing the feet may assist in tolerating the cold.

Alternating hot and cold showers change the distribution of blood throughout the entire body. Blood is pulled from the internal organs to the skin. Showers give a mechanical stimulation that tub baths do not provide.

The salt glow skin rub is often invigorating. Stand in a tub of hot water. Moisten the hands and body with water, dip hands into a container of salt, and rub the skin briskly. Shower to remove salt from the skin.

The cold mitten friction is carried out by wringing washcloths or mitts from ice water and briskly rubbing the body, refreshing the cloths as they warm up. Start at the head and progress downward toward the feet. The body should be warm before treatment is begun.

Abdominal cold packs and cold showers have been shown more effective in relieving fatigue than rest. Blood pulled from other parts of the body bring glucose, oxygen, and other fatigue-relieving substances into the area. Temperatures of the cold packs ranged from 45 to 50 degrees F. Cold packs were left in place for ten minutes. Showers consisted of ten minute sprays at 55 to 60 degrees F. to the trunk.

Heating treatments are helpful for those suffering from chronic fatigue, but should not be prolonged. Prolonged heat has a depressing effect, which worsens fatigue. Five to six minutes may be sufficient to start vigorous sweating, then the treatment should be concluded with a cold treatment--a cold shower, cold towel rub, wet sheet rub, or salt glow. The purpose of the treatment is to stimulate circulation and toxin elimination from the skin.

Outdoor life is beneficial to the fatigue sufferer. Breathing devitalized, deoxygenated indoor air deprives the body of oxygen.

Respiratory exercises are often helpful in increasing energy levels. While walking, try to inhale for five steps, then exhale for six steps, Take slow, deep breaths, attempting to fill and empty the lungs as completely as possible.

Another method of exercising the lungs is to take a deep breath and read out loud as long as possible with that single breath. With time the lung capacity will increase.

Drugs are not the solution to fatigue. Many physicians automatically give a person complaining of fatigue sedatives or antidepressants, which only compound the problem.

CHRONIC FATIGUE SYNDROME

Chronic fatigue syndrome, also called "yuppie flu," myalgic encephalomyelitis, chronic fatigue immune dysfunction syndrome, post infection chronic fatigue, chronic Epstein-Barr virus syndrome, and chronic mononucleosis syndrome, has only recently been classified as a disease. The cause is not clearly understood. It is probably the disease called "neurasthenia" in the 1860's, anemia, hypoglycemia, environmental allergy or candidiasis down through the ages. Some feel it is due to an infection by the Epstein-Barr virus, a common virus to which most Americans have been exposed. The majority of these patients have been observed to have allergies, which suggests the possibility that it could be a hypersensitive immune system reaction. Other researchers feel that a Herpes-virus Type 6 may be the causative agent. Chronic fatigue syndrome may also be another manifestation of the fibrositis syndrome. A California researcher suggests an association with rubella immunizations, and calls for further research in this area.

The true incidence is not known, but chronic fatigue is said to be the seventh most common complaint heard by family physicians.

Chronic fatigue syndrome came to the attention of the public in 1985, with the outbreak of a strange fatigue-associated cluster of symptoms which occurred in the Lake Tahoe, Nevada region. A group of scientists from Centers for Disease Control, the National Cancer Institute, and Harvard University, went to the area to try to determine the cause. By 1987 more than 200 cases had been identified in the area. Most of the patients were young, female, and highly educated.

Overwhelming fatigue is often the primary symptom. Sufferers wake up exhausted despite a long night of sleep, and can hardly stay awake during the day. They may have swollen, tender lymph glands, achiness, sleep disturbances, memory and concentration disruptions, depression, headache, low-grade fever, sore throat, weakness, joint and muscle pains. Some complain of bladder problems, numbness, enlarged spleen or liver, eyelid swelling, nausea, diarrhea, neck pain, coldness of extremities, ringing in the ears, muscle twitches, clumsiness, shivering, shortness of breath, abdominal cramping, weight loss or gain, skin rash, fast heart rate, chest pain, light sensitivity, irritability, cough, dizziness, blurred vision, and night sweats. Symptoms vary in intensity from day to day, and throughout the day. Onset is often with flu-like disease such as flu or mononucleosis, or viral disease such as bronchitis, hepatitis, or gastrointestinal disease. These symptoms persist even after the associated disease would be expected to be gone.

Diagnosis is elusive as there is no definitive test available. Diagnosis is made primarily by eliminating other causes of fatigue. M e d i c a l science currently has no recognized treatment, but there are effective home remedies and lifestyle changes which many have found beneficial or curative. The patient must take the primary responsibility for his health care. Rest must be balanced by exercise, the diet must be carefully regulated, and excessive and prolonged stress should be avoided. Symptoms sometimes remit, or may wax and wane over the course of a year. Recovery may occur over a period of years, with setbacks from infections or over-exertion.

TREATMENT:

Many chronic fatigue syndrome patients report that standing in one position is more tiring than walking. When standing, shift the weight frequently, and sing, whistle or sigh deeply through pursed lips to encourage deep breathing. If the legs are tired after activities, attention should be directed toward activities involving arm movement.

The diet should be low in fat, and high in unrefined carbohydrates. Physical endurance has been shown to be decreased on a high fat diet. Eliminate all free fats (fats added to foods in preparation, or at the table). The nutrition rule to follow is to eat freely of fruits, vegetables and whole grains. Anything else would be added sparingly, if at all. That would call for the sparing use of salt, sugar, honey, nutritional supplements of all kinds, nutritional yeast, etc. We recommend the complete elimination of all free fats (margarine, mayonnaise, cheese, fried foods, cooking fats, salad oils and butter made from nuts and seeds (peanut butter, tahini, etc.), spices, (ginger, cinnamon, nutmeg, cloves, black and red pepper, allspice), baking soda and powder.

Many people with chronic fatigue syndrome have associated allergies. Those who suffer from food allergies will be benefited by a diet free of the foods they are sensitive to. Most common food allergens reported by chronic fatigue syndrome sufferers include milk, eggs, chocolate, coffee, red wine, and cereal grains (wheat, corn, barley, rye, and oats. Rice and millet may be tolerated). Elimination of the food for four to six weeks may produce improvement in symptoms. For more information on food allergies see our book, *Food Allergies Made Simple*. People with food allergies often crave the very foods they are sensitive to.

Other allergens known to induce fatigue include cosmetics, perfumes, hair sprays, soaps, bubble baths, toothpaste, nicotine, and gas fumes.

Foods should be eaten in as near a natural state as possible, with minimal preparation. A good variety of fruits, vegetables and whole grains is the diet of choice. Fried and rich foods, spices, chocolate, tobacco, and alcohol should be eliminated. Many benefit from a dairy free diet. Meals should be eaten slowly, and thoroughly chewed. Unchewed food particles place an additional burden on the digestive system.

Food should be taken only at mealtimes; eating between meals forces the digestive system to work when it should have opportunity to rest. Suppers taken late in the day force the digestive system to work during the night hours. Breakfast should be hearty, lunch substantial, and supper, if eaten, light and early.

Fasting one day a week, with the intake of plenty of pure, fresh water, may be helpful.

Caffeine, found in many beverages, medications, and chocolate, should be eliminated as it may interfere with sleep. Caffeine and other naturally occurring chemicals in coffee, tea, and colas are often in themselves a cause of fatigue.

A sufficient fluid intake is essential to the elimination of fatigue. Thirst is not an adequate guide to water requirements. Fluid intake should be enough to replace fluids lost, and to keep the urine pale in color at all times. Water is the beverage of choice.

Sugar, which is stimulating, should be avoided. A study comparing the effectiveness of a sugar snack and a brisk 10 minute walk in the treatment of fatigue demonstrated greater fatigue relief from the walk! Those who took the sugar snack initially had increased energy, but one hour later had increased fatigue and lowered energy levels.

Some with chronic fatigue syndrome also have Candida infection. A two week trial of yeast-free foods may result in improvement. Avoid baked goods made with yeast, juices, mushrooms, vitamin B supplements, dried fruits and aged or fermented foods such as vinegar, cheese, malted foods, liquor, beer, or wine.

Constipation should be carefully guarded against by the intake of adequate fluids and fiber.

Regularity in bed and rising times assists the body in learning to sleep on schedule. If extra rest is needed the person should rise at the regular time, then return to bed later in the day, but never after meals as that can cause fat plugging of tiny arteries in the heart. An irregular schedule is known to induce fatigue, as manifested by jet lag. Afternoon naps may interfere with night sleep.

Give attention to proper breathing habits. Good posture, and respirations from the abdomen rather than the chest are essential to proper ventilation. Do deep breathing exercises two or three times a day, and during periods of stress. Consider taking lessons in singing or speech to develop the diaphragm.

Refuse to give in to the disease process. Exercise should be done to tolerance on a regular schedule. Exercise helps depression, and improves oxygenation of the blood, which is essential to energy. The exercise should be something you really enjoy doing, as enthusiasm will permit one to exercise for longer periods. Avoid competitive activities, as they are stressful. Exercise stimulates the body to produce endorphins which fight fatigue and elevate the mood. It will also promote better sleep. Sleep before midnight is more likely to result in production of growth hormone which gives ambition and energy to adults. Try a 9:00 P.M. bedtime.

Alcohol and sleeping pills disrupt the normal sleep cycles and should be avoided. Immunizations should be avoided. As a general rule all drugs encourage fatigue.

Vitamin supplements are often recommended, but these place an additional burden on the body as it must eliminate the excess. Most nutrients have a see-saw relationship with each other. By taking one essential nutrient as a supplement you may depress another equally essential nutrient.

Overweight fatigue sufferers should reduce their weight to normal or slightly below. The heart must pump blood through three-fourths of a mile of extra blood vessels for every pound the body is overweight.

Fever is the body's method of fighting infection. Hot baths (101-102 degrees F.) may be used for 20-30 minutes once daily to produce an artificial fever, which will stimulate the immune system. Apply cold cloths wrung from ice water to the face or head to keep the head cool when the mouth temperature goes above 100 degrees. An alternate method, especially for younger, reasonably healthy persons, is to use a water temperature of 108-110 degrees F. to raise oral temperature to 103-104 degrees F. It is well to have an attendant for this method. (See the book *Home Remedies* for details of treatment.)

Several lifestyle change centers, among them Uchee Pines Institute in Seale, Alabama, and Poland Spring Institute, Poland Spring, Maine, have had excellent results in the chronic fatigue syndrome. They have used full-body hyperthermia utilizing the heated whirlpool or Russian steam bath and have incorporated the lifestyle changes previously mentioned. Hyperthermia treatments have averaged 10-20, given at daily intervals, with oral temperatures usually reaching 103-104 degrees F.

Steps should be taken to strengthen the immune system. Elimination of toxins (alcohol, tobacco, medications, allergens) is essential. Out-of-doors exercise, and sun exposure are advisable. Sun early or late in the day.

Gargling with warm salt water and a heating compress to the throat may bring relief for sore throats. Chronic sore throat is a good sign of food sensitivity. Try to discover what the food is by selective elimination of a group of foods. If the sore throat goes away, add back one food at a time every five days.

Joint pains (also a sign of food sensitivity) can often be relieved with the use of either hot or cold applications. Use whichever produces the most benefit.

Liver involvement may be treated by hot compresses over the upper right portion of the abdomen for twenty minutes twice a day.

INDEX